I0114177

— HOW TO —
PROTECT
YOUR LIFE
SAVINGS
— FROM —
NURSING HOMES

HOW TO
PROTECT
YOUR LIFE
SAVINGS
FROM
NURSING HOMES

A SIMPLE, ACTIONABLE GUIDE to SHIELD YOUR ASSETS from LONG-TERM CARE COSTS

JOSHUA RAE

Walnut Limited

York, PA

Contents

Chapter 5

If You're More Than Five Years Away from Assisted Living,

Chapter 6

This book is for informational purposes only. It is not intended to serve as a substitute for professional advice. The author and publisher specifically disclaim any and all liability arising directly or indirectly from the use of any information contained in this book. A professional should be consulted regarding your specific situation. Any product mentioned in this book does not imply endorsement of that product by the author or publisher.

The conversations in the book are based on the author's recollections, though they are not intended to represent word-for-word transcripts. Rather, the author has retold them in a way that communicates the meaning of what was said. In the author's humble opinion, the essence of the dialogue is accurate in all instances.

How to Protect Your Life Savings from Nursing Homes copyright © 2022 by Joshua Rae

All rights reserved. No part of this book may be used or reproduced in any manner whatsoever without written permission of the publisher, except in the case of brief quotations embodied in critical articles or reviews.

Walnut Limited
340 Imperial Drive
York PA 17403
nursinghometrusts.org
Send feedback to josh@nursinghometrusts.org

Publisher's Cataloging-In-Publication Data
    Names: Rae, Joshua, author.
    Title: How to protect your life savings from nursing homes : a simple, actionable guide to shield your
assets from long-term care costs / Joshua Rae.
    Description: York, PA : Walnut Limited, [2022]
    Identifiers: ISBN: 979-8-9867788-0-8 (hardcover) | 979-8-9867788-1-5 (softcover) |
979-8-9867788-2-2 (ebook) | 979-8-9867788-3-9 (audiobook)
    Subjects: LCSH: Older people--Finance, Personal. | Older people--Long-term care--United
States--Planning. | Estate planning--United States. | Nursing homes--United States--Costs. |
Medicaid.
    Classification: LCC: HG179 .R34 2022 | DDC: 332.02400846--dc23

Special discounts for bulk sales are available.
Please contact josh@nursinghometrusts.org

To my grandmas:
May your end-of-life experiences help all those who read this.

Tell Me What You Think

Let other readers know what you thought of *How to Protect Your Life Savings from Nursing Homes*. Please write an honest review for this book on your favorite online bookshop.

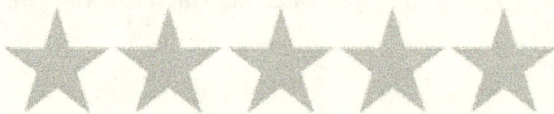

★★★★★

What Happens When You Visit www.nursinghometrusts.org?

First, you'll notice the "How Much Can I Protect?" button on our site. That button will take you to an estimator that calculates how much you can protect by following the strategies in this book. It takes only five minutes.

Once you get your protection estimate, we'll invite you to book a free consultation with one of our licensed representatives. During that call, we'll let you know in exact terms how we can help you. It may take only a digital signature on some paperwork that costs you nothing.

If you're in crisis planning mode and your loved one is already in a nursing home, spending down is necessary right now. Depending on how many children your loved ones have and their total assets, a funeral expense trust for Mom and burial space item trusts for the kids may be enough to spend down completely. Then all the money will be protected when Mom applies for Medicaid. Once she's accepted, you're in the clear.

Maybe your loved one has a home and needs to sell it. Or you have a lot of money, and you want to set up a single premium immediate annuity in conjunction with an elder care attorney. We'll work on that project together and get an attorney in the mix.

Or maybe you're planning well in advance and just need an attorney to establish some trusts. Whatever you need for your current situation, we'll be ready to assist you.

Now is the time to protect your family legacy. Visit www.nursinghometrusts.org and set up your free consultation with us.

CHAPTER 1

•

HOW TO KEEP YOUR MONEY

A woman I'd never met before handed me $95,000 at a coffee shop. One of the earliest life savings protection cases I'd worked on was with an attorney named Steve Brown. Steve had been charged with caring for one particular woman's **estate** and was working with the woman's daughter, Sarah. (Please see the **Glossary** for more details about words in boldface.) Sarah's mom—Henrietta—had dementia and was living out her days in a nursing home. Steve referred the case to me.

Over several phone calls, I learned that Henrietta had $120,000 total left in her various accounts. She had already lost tens of thousands to pay for the nursing home, and over the next several months, that facility would spend down the rest of it—all $120,000. Until the elderly woman was left with empty accounts. Nothing. Decades of making frugal decisions, clipping coupons, and saving diligently would be erased in a year or less.

In the United States, financial destitution on paper triggers **Medic-aid**, the federal program that covers health care expenses of impoverished individuals living in nursing homes. Medicaid does not cover nursing home costs for residents with means. Only after a patient's financial legacy is totally gone—covering nursing home expenses—can federal money reimburse the nursing home for care.

Unless you act fast.

That was Sarah's situation. She and her four other siblings knew little about estate planning, but they knew enough to hope that someone could shield Mom's life savings from the nursing home *and* allow Medicaid to cover her expenses. It sounds complicated because it is. But with time ticking, Sarah had to make a decision. And that decision was giving a complete stranger almost $100,000 over a cup of coffee. The money would be lost if she didn't.

Sarah, as the oldest of her siblings, knew her mom's financial fate was in her hands. Sadly, Henrietta's mind was gone. As is typical with advanced dementia, she didn't recognize her family anymore, not even her beloved firstborn daughter. However, Henrietta had two facts in her favor—she was in good physical health, and she would live a *long* time. Years, possibly. But long-term care expenses require immediate-term actions.

That day at our local coffee shop, Sarah entrusted me with $95,000 worth of checks to establish **trusts** for her, her siblings, and all their spouses. She decided to do this, despite knowing that I was a young, new-to-the-industry insurance professional who had never before set up **irrevocable trusts** for anyone. That was the depth of Henrietta's financial crisis. Even my employer, Golden Considerations, was new to working with the general public on trusts. We were already the nation's leading independent broker of funeral expense insurance trusts, with over $100 million in annual client premiums, but at the time, we were purely a business-to-business company and didn't serve people like Sarah directly. It was this meeting in a coffee shop that opened my eyes. Shortly after this meeting, we launched www.nursinghometrusts.org to assist clients like Sarah across the whole country.

Assist her, we did. The checks Sarah gave me at that coffee shop came from three sources—Henrietta's savings, the value of a **whole life insurance** policy, and cash from Henrietta's old car that Sarah and her siblings had sold. By trusting us, that family ultimately kept $95,000 instead of zero.

I wrote this book to show you how any American can get Medicaid to pay for some or all long-term care expenses without wasting time, losing money, or getting overcharged by a nursing home motivated by profit first. To show you how, let's begin with what I told Sarah in a subsequent conversation where we discussed the difference between

Medicaid, the federal assistance program, and the better-known health care agency Medicare.

Medicare, Medicaid, and Paying Nursing Homes without Going Broke

First, let's clarify the difference between Medicare and Medicare. **Medicare** is a health insurance program provided by the US government. Every citizen over age sixty-five receives Medicare benefits, as well as entitlements like Social Security. Medicaid is a needs-based program that requires your family member to be impoverished to qualify.

When your loved one enters a nursing home, Medicare pays for up to three months of care. After that final month of Medicare compensation, things get . . . crazy. Unless you have **long-term care insurance** (sometimes called LTC), your loved one must pay out-of-pocket before they are Medicaid-eligible. LTC used to be common, but with longer life spans and rising health care costs, LTC is out of most families' ranges. Once you are off Medicare, you have to pay approximately $10,000 per month out-of-pocket until the program classifies you as "impoverished." In most US states, that means nursing home residents have less than $2,000 in assets (some have $0), excluding their home and car. Only then can they apply for Medicaid, which pays for care until death—well, sort of. I'll explain this shortly.

Earlier, I said *up to three months* because not everybody qualifies for three full months of Medicare coverage—or one hundred days, to be precise—when they find themselves in a nursing home. The following four statements must be true for Medicare to cover the stay:

1. The patient had a three-day minimum inpatient hospital stay that was deemed medically necessary (not including the discharge date);
2. The patient was admitted to the nursing home within thirty days of hospital discharge;

3. The patient needs daily skilled nursing or rehabilitation care for the reason they were hospitalized in the first place; and
4. The patient received a physician's referral or other order deeming that nursing home care was necessary.

Even if someone qualifies, Medicare doesn't cover everything. Patients still must submit a copay from day twenty-one of their nursing home state onward. Patient only receives complete Medicare coverage for days one through twenty—and that's if the above four statements are true. After that, from day twenty-one through one hundred, patients must pay $194.50 per day for their stay.

Let's say an elderly neighbor undergoes hip replacement surgery but suffers an infection that lands her in the hospital for five days. She is discharged from the hospital to a local nursing home for daily rehabilitation and skilled nursing to prevent reinfection. Your neighbor needs four weeks—twenty-eight days—of care. Days twenty-one through twenty-eight require a daily $194.50 copay, so her Medicare bill on the date of discharge from the nursing home is $1,556.

That's a far cry from *up to three months of Medicare coverage*, I'll admit. If your neighbor is unable to recover enough to return home and must receive nursing home care long term, the bad news gets worse.

Now, that $1,556 is peanuts compared to the impending spending. Once Medicare stops paying and copaying, your neighbor starts paying—and pays and pays, until she is impoverished and can finally qualify for Medicaid. The time between these programs is most important for your neighbor—where she loses it all or protects what she's allowed. It happens fast, at a rate of $10,000 a month.

Once your neighbor is "spent down," "impoverished," and enrolled in Medicaid, the program tallies everything they pay the nursing home until she passes away. This explains my "sort of" earlier. After death, if there's no living spouse, Medicaid hits the deceased's estate for any assets left behind, like a house or car, to claw back as much of what Medicaid paid as possible. Every day, financial legacies are obliterated across the country in this manner. No money, no house, no car . . . nothing for the kids and grandkids.

Why the System Leaves You With Nothing (And What to Do About It)

There is no free lunch. There is no free long-term care.

In the United States, the federal health care assistance system is built by design to leave you and your family with nothing. Every generation is forced to start from zero. Even if you do everything right—you plan for the future, you set aside savings—the system is out to get you. If you drank or gambled away your wealth, the system rewards you. You've already impoverished yourself, so Medicaid welcomes you into their program right away. But if you worked hard, hoping to leave a legacy for your kids and grandkids, the vultures come for you. They'll tear you apart until there's nothing left.

This is a mass exploitation of humans in our most vulnerable state. Not only does Grandma or Dad or your husband not remember you anymore due to dementia, but the nursing home adds ruin to the pain. They seize everything, spending it all until you're depleted to $2,000 or less. Then they take the house back in the asset recovery period while the whole family is still grieving, demanding that you now sell the family farm.

This book will help you prevent these nightmares. I had to write this book because it didn't exist. No other guide to long-term care planning is written—and priced—with the average person in mind. There are five-hundred-page reference manuals and dense legal textbooks, but no easy reads that deliver immediate results.

I wrote this book to help you make dramatic, positive changes to how you approach long-term and end-of-life care for yourself and your family. Most people think of a nursing home as the last place they would want to leave their loved ones. Regardless of staff, amenities, or overall quality, they feel like the nursing home is out to get them. COVID-19 made that perception worse. Many clients of ours were prohibited from seeing their parents and spouses during the pandemic; most nursing homes in the United States banned visitation. One woman brought a ladder to her mom's nursing home so they could discuss at the window what she was doing to protect her wealth.

Even so, I do want to clarify that nursing homes aren't necessarily "the bad guy" in all stories about long-term care and legacy. Nursing home accountants simply don't care where the money comes from. It's all the same to them whether they're taking Mom's last penny or federal Medicaid checks.

What nursing homes hate is the transition from private pay to public pay. They want to make sure your Medicaid application is approved. If the transition isn't done right, and the Medicaid application fails after the patient is spent down, the nursing home is hung out to dry because the private money is gone, and the public money isn't flowing yet.

Nursing homes work to prevent or mitigate the friction caused by changing funding sources. They have entire departments built around "revenue cycle management." Whether you're on Medicaid or paying out-of-pocket doesn't matter to them as long as the money keeps flowing.

Nursing homes won't tell you these harsh truths. One of the only asset protection techniques they do tell you about is funeral planning. They don't want children to abandon their parents in nursing homes just because the kids don't want to pay for their funerals. If that happens, the nursing home is stuck with the body, and unfortunately, this isn't uncommon. So, nursing homes will advocate for you to plan and fund the funeral, but that's all they will reveal.

One of our clients came to us to set up a funeral plan for her mom. They were two years into a Medicaid **spend-down period**, and the nursing home had already burned through $200,000 of their money. We were looking at their last $5,000. If she'd gotten expert advice two years prior, the majority of that wealth would have been preserved.

The harsh reality is that this happens all the time. These stories may be hard to read, but this book will not sugarcoat reality. It will teach you how to prevent these financial tragedies.

This Book Is for You If . . .

This book is for people with a loved one who is in a nursing home or soon to be in one. You stay up at night thinking about your loved one's health and the insane cost of care. You have a haunting feeling that they're going to lose everything . . . and you are right to worry.

Let's assume you are looking after your parent, grandparent, or spouse. If you go into this environment ignorant of these harsh realities, it's like walking into the open jaws of a hungry beast.

If you have an elder care attorney to handle advance planning, awesome—but the vast majority of people don't. My book is not for multimillionaires who have had lawyers on their payroll for decades. Those people don't need my help.

This book is for average Americans who have paid taxes and now need care. It will teach you how to protect your family's nest egg. After reading my book, you will know how to protect your family's life savings from the vultures waiting to take it all.

This book will help you help your kids so they don't have to start from scratch. They can get a head start with the legacy you have worked so hard to leave them.

You need someone to tell you the truth. If you have been through the nursing home process, you know how high the paperwork is stacked. It's bewildering. This book will bring you relief. It will help you navigate the tough situations you are likely to face with rich, actionable advice. This book will give realistic examples that connect readers emotionally. Not just cold facts, laws, and statistics.

There are not many worse feelings than feeling like a sucker. Learn to preserve your wealth so it goes to family and charity, not nursing homes and the government. My book shows you how.

If your loved one is in a nursing home, the cost of inaction is about $300 per day taken from your loved one's estate—from your family inheritance. That's $2,100 a week, or over $8,000 a month.

Let that sink in. **Every day you delay reading and finishing this book costs your loved one $300.**

If someone in your family is in or nearing a nursing home situation, it could cost your family everything if you do not act. And you can act! You can protect the savings your family spent a lifetime building. You only need the right information.

But it is almost impossible to find the information you need by your-self—even on the internet! Families run into walls of indecipherable Medicaid bylaws. If you are lucky, you can find a competent attorney who will charge you $10,000 to $20,000 for the right to hear information that should be easy to find.

I can give you that priceless information because I have spent my entire career in the senior planning and care industry. I have watched for more than fifteen years as families have struggled to find and process the information they need to plan effectively.

And the clock is ticking. The Baby Boom generation is hitting retirement age. More people than ever stand to benefit over the next several years. Now is the time to learn this information. Here's where to start.

How to Get the Most from This Book

This book is written to address different scenarios. Depending on your situation, the decisions you make could either secure your family's life savings or cause massive headaches.

For example, if you're a healthy person that wrote your son a $100,000 check, or if you placed your home in your daughter's name, you might be free and clear. But if you did these same actions within five years of applying for Medicaid (and were found otherwise eligible), you'll trigger a **penalty period**. Medicaid will not pay for anything during that penalty period, starting from the date you applied for coverage.

Each chapter in the book is designed for a specific situation. While each chapter has value for everybody, if you are in a desperate situation, read the chapter that applies to you, and follow its advice.

- If the nursing home already ate your estate, I'm sorry . . . there is nothing we can do to help.
- If you or a loved one is currently in or about to be in a nursing home, read **Chapter 2**.
- Is your loved one new to a nursing home and in the first three months of Medicare or long-term care insurance? Read **Chapter 3**.

- If your loved one might need a nursing home in less than five years, read **Chapter 4**.
- If your loved one might need a nursing home after five or more years, read **Chapter 5**.
- If you're in family law, wealth management, or a related profession, read *all* chapters to better understand how to guide your clients.

Maybe you have multiple family members at different life stages. Perhaps your ailing spouse may need long-term care soon, your dad might need long-term care in a decade or more, and you also want to protect your money for your own kids. Read *all* the chapters.

Time is money. Get the exact information you need right now, and act quickly. Remember, inaction costs $300 a day.

So, are you ready to take the next step? Flip to the chapter that best suits your needs. Protecting your legacy—and your posterity—starts here.

CHAPTER 2

•

IF THE NURSING HOME IS EATING YOUR ESTATE RIGHT NOW, READ THIS

Author's Note: The content of this chapter is specifically for readers who are already in a nursing home and will likely be staying long term, as well as their loved ones. The Medicaid spend-down period has already begun; the patient's estate is being liquidated. Other readers may find this material insightful or useful.

"The nursing home will take everything. There's nothing you can do."

Nursing homes are a $197 billion industry because millions of families believe this. They have resigned themselves to the fact that if the nursing home wants Dad's life savings, they are going to get it, and nothing can be done. Dad's assets can't be moved, can't be given away, can't be saved. But it's simply not true—Dad's financial legacy can be saved.

Every week, I get calls from funeral directors, attorneys, and financial advisors with referrals to people they think we can help.

"I've got a client here. We just did a funeral expense trust for her," they'll say. "She's got a hundred thousand dollars left in savings. She needs to talk with you."

One such referral was for a ninety-three-year-old woman I'll call Theresa, residing in a suburban Pennsylvania assisted living community. She was blessed with unusually good health and a strong mind, but Theresa's kids believed she might need a wheelchair over the next few weeks to stay mobile. That would mark the great transition out of assisted living and into a nursing home, and in turn, a huge increase in cost.

Medicaid almost never covers any assisted living costs. Even though a nursing home costs significantly more than assisted living when you pay out-of-pocket, Medicaid can cover almost all nursing home costs—*if you qualify*. I wrote this book because for most people, what it takes to qualify for Medicaid is financial catastrophe. You must be broke (fewer than $2,000 to your name) in order for Medicaid to cover your nursing home expenses. Thus, Medicaid requires your savings, income, and assets be spent down or seized until you have only $2,000 left; then and only then will Medicaid help.

That was about to be Theresa's story. She told me over the phone that she had no house but just over $100,000 in savings. The nursing home's business office manager led her family to believe their mother was not allowed to do anything with her money—and that it would soon be theirs.

I encouraged Theresa to invite her daughter Rachel to our phone appointment, because all relevant family members should be involved when making elder care decisions. Much like her mother, Rachel was sharp. My first task was to dispel the misconception that they could not protect Mom's money from the nursing home.

"We can protect more money?" Theresa asked.

"Yes, you can," I said. "Even given the Medicaid rules about giving money to kids and spending down a senior's estate."

"But the nursing home said they will be taking all of Mom's money," Rachel said.

"Yes and no," I said. "You can't just hide it in a checking or savings account. And you can't give it to charity, much less to family members.

But you can protect at least half. Maybe more. But this has to be done with specific legal requirements in mind, which I'll tell you about."

"Please do!" Theresa and Rachel said in unison.

Now I'll tell you.

There Is Hope

Nursing home costs are outrageous. Every month, nursing homes drain an average of $8,365 from 1.4 million innocent seniors. Every year, nursing homes force thousands of families into **bankruptcy** and poverty. Lives and legacies are ruined by a system that fails to provide for senior citizens when they need help the most. If you're in this situation, Medicare isn't helping anymore, if it ever did.

People are told they cannot do anything with Mom or Dad's money because doing so disqualifies them from Medicaid. They're told not to give money away or accept any from their loved ones. Otherwise, it will trigger a penalty period, and their loved ones will lose everything through private pay. Then *they* will have to keep paying after the money runs out.

Even if you know what to do, the paperwork is a nightmare. You must grant nursing homes access to bank accounts, assign Social Security payments, and untangle miles of red tape. If you thought signing a mortgage was bad, this is ten times worse.

Don't expect help from the nursing home. Their business office is there to look out for *their* financial interests, not yours. Whether it comes from private pay or Medicaid, the business office's job is to make sure the money keeps flowing. That's why nursing homes will advise patients' families to prefund funerals before they go on Medicaid: they don't want to fund burials themselves.

And the business office tracks every last cent of a patient's money. That way they can drain the patient's accounts to almost nothing. Then Medicaid kicks in. The nursing home also *prefers* out-of-pocket payments instead of Medicaid because the facility earns significantly more from private pay than public funds. Allegedly, nursing homes charge patients as much as 40 percent *more* for identical care when patients or their families pay directly.

Well, maybe. Maybe not, you might think. Maybe you're not worried right now. Perhaps your mom has $50,000 left in her account.

That's only five or six months of care. It's better for the nursing home to say nothing during the spend-down period so your mom becomes impoverished. Then they'll say they need you to sign up for Medicaid to cover Mom's continuing expenses.

They won't advocate for your best interests or give you options. They'll wait. Meanwhile, they'll determine your overall financial picture to ensure you're ready for Medicaid once you're poor. After your loved one passes away, Medicaid will feast on what's left of the estate.

It doesn't have to be this way. What you'll learn in this chapter and throughout this book are practical, legal strategies and tools our clients deploy every day to protect tens of thousands of dollars in life savings and future inheritances. And that's not to mention how you can save your loved one's dignity and your family's peace of mind.

Feel free to take a break from this book at any time to visit www. nursinghometrusts.org for more information.

No, the nursing home won't look out for you. But you can look out for yourself. In this chapter, we'll cover how you can protect your home and your cash.

How to Protect Your Home

A home is your family's greatest asset. You need to protect it. That's not easy. People often believe assets like homes are safe, but they're often in jeopardy unless someone takes action. The patient's family can indeed keep the home. The approach the family can use depends on whether the patient is single or married.

If your loved one is married with a community spouse, then the home is safe. A **community spouse** is any spouse who lives in the community and is not in a nursing home or receiving Medicaid. When a patient (or an institutionalized spouse) goes into a nursing home, a community spouse gets to keep the family home, even after their loved one in the nursing home dies. To put it simply, if someone enters a nursing home and their spouse is still living in the community, their spouse can almost always keep the home with no further repercussions. Note that this does not apply to second homes.

But what about Grandma who lived at home alone before entering the nursing home?

Most nursing homes tell patients and their families that they can keep the home, even if they're single (typically, up to a house value of $595,000). However, after Grandma applies for Medicaid, families are not aware of what happens next. That's when the nursing home keeps a tally of all the resources they've spent on Grandma via Medicaid until she passes away. Afterward, Medicaid comes for the deceased's estate. In most states nationwide, Medicaid will go after the home because it is normally part of the estate.

That grandma example is typical of most financial situations involving a single or widowed individual. To return to the earlier point, when a nursing home tells a patient's family they can keep their home, they most likely mean that the family can keep the home *for now*. Few realize that Medicaid payments to the nursing home on the patient's behalf are a debt that must be paid as much as possible during the estate recovery period. Just as there's no free lunch, there's no free nursing home.

If you're in this position, with no community spouse, your options are limited. But that doesn't mean you have none. Here's how you can protect your loved one's home.

Transfer the Home

Gifting a home to someone normally triggers a Medicaid penalty period. However, there are three exceptions.

The first exception is that the admitting patient can always give the house to a child under twenty-one years of age, a child who is blind, or a child who is permanently disabled. This triggers no penalty periods.

The second exception is for an adult child who lived in the home and provided care to their father or mother for two years prior to entering the nursing home. The government views this as the child saving them two years of Medicaid bills, so they let them have the home as thanks.

The third exception is gifting the house to any sibling of the individual in the nursing home as long as the sibling:

- Has **equity** interest in the home (ownership of as little as 1 percent); or
- Has lived in the home for at least a year prior to the nursing home admission date.

This will also be relevant in the next chapter. If a nursing home is on the horizon but not imminent, you can deed a small percentage of your home to a sibling and move them in. As long as the sibling pays market price for that 1 percent, there is no penalty period. After a year, you can be admitted to the nursing home and transfer the home fully to the sibling without penalty.

What if none of these apply to your situation, but you don't want to lose the family home?

Sell the home to a family member. But not for $1. It must be for what's considered "a reasonable market price." Hire a professional appraiser, or go off the assessed tax value, then multiply that by the **common level ratio**.

The home sale generates income, which will disqualify your loved one from Medicaid coverage until the cash is spent down on nursing home fees **or protected**. *Then* the patient can reapply for Medicaid.

In my own family's case, our Western Pennsylvania home was worth $100,000. But after multiplying it by the common level ratio, we got an assessed value of $87,000. My cousin will buy the home from my grandma for $87,000, and then we'll protect the money from the sale with specialized irrevocable trusts. (I'll explain more about this shortly.) Grandma will apply for a home **waiver** program, which is like Medicaid for home care—it helps people stay in their homes instead of in a nursing home. The program will send nurses several times a week to provide in-home care. Meanwhile, Grandma will pay rent to my cousin, and the $87,000 will be protected.

It's a complicated process. But it's necessary in this day and age. I'm here to guide you through it.

There are several other important resources for people who don't fall into these three exception categories and for whom selling a home to a family member isn't an option. These resources will still help you keep a home you would otherwise lose in estate recovery after a family member in a nursing home passes away. They are:

1. **Transfers for exclusively non-Medicaid purposes:** If you can show with objective evidence that you transferred the home without regard to Medicaid planning (you can't fake this), then it's exempt. Let's say you legitimately gave the home to a family member (who doesn't fit any of the above three exceptions) three years ago because you wanted to rent a small apartment. You also can prove that you had no knowledge about going into a nursing home; maybe an unexpected Alzheimer's diagnosis changed everyone's plans. Then you can exempt this transaction from being a gift that triggers a penalty period. You'll likely need to hire an attorney.

2. **Undue hardship claim:** The family can file this claim during estate recovery of the home. An undue hardship claim might be that seizing a working farm would be so unprofitable that it would put the family out of business. Again, expect to hire an attorney.

Next, let's look at ways to protect your home and car.

Consider Home (and Car) Upgrades

You can also upgrade your home to protect your estate. Let's say a married couple owns a fully paid-off home worth $250,000, and they have another $250,000 in savings. The husband goes to a nursing home while the wife stays in the family home.

The law says that if a spouse goes into a nursing home, the community spouse gets to keep a certain amount of money. (This is known as the Community Spouse Resource Allowance; more on this later.) Everything above and beyond that threshold gets spent down, or the nursing home can seize it.

In this example, the wife could take the money and upgrade the home. She could redo the bathroom to make it accessible, put in new flooring, build a wheelchair ramp for the main door, and make other repairs. She is allowed by law to put money into one house.

The community spouse is also allowed one car. What kind doesn't matter, within restrictions. It could be a Fiat or a Range Rover. She could sell the old car and buy a nice new one as long as it's not a classic antique, like an original Model T, or an investment-grade purchase, like a Lamborghini.

Compare that to what happens if the person has no living community spouse. Home improvements and a car upgrade might be nice ways to delay the nursing home spend down, but Medicaid may still seize those assets during estate recovery to pay down debts after your loved one's death.

Inventory Personal Effects

Personal effects do not count against you as assets. So while you're renovating (or cleaning out) the family home, pay special attention to these. Personal effects include jewelry, clothing, personal care items, musical instruments, and hobby items.

If Grandma is on Medicaid now and buys $100,000 worth of jewelry at Tiffany's, that will raise a huge red flag. But personal effects she owned before applying for Medicaid can be passed on without issue.

How to Protect Your Cash

Whether the home stays in the family or not, the sale will generate cash. Maybe the home was sold years ago, and the family member has been in assisted living or renting an apartment.

Regardless of the situation, your family member will show up in the nursing home with cash. It could be in checking, savings, retirement accounts, or a whole life, universal life, or final expense insurance policy. Those need to be spent down before the person can apply for Medicaid.

I specialize in helping clients who fall into this category. However, protecting their money isn't as straightforward as transferring it from one account to another. You can't *just* accept money from your loved one.

In fact, the worst thing you can do in this situation is give away money. In general, any transactions in your savings or credit account over $500 in the last five years are scrutinized during the Medicaid **look-back period**. Even one could trigger a penalty period.

If you just take or give away cash, Medicaid will flag that transfer and penalize you. They will refuse to pay for your family member's care until the penalty period is over. (See the **Appendix** for state-specific penalty period calculation instructions.)

These penalty periods represent the worst-case scenario for a nursing home—providing care without compensation. Caring for a patient costs a lot, and the money has to come from somewhere. In most cases, the law doesn't make the kids pay, and it is not easy for the nursing home to legally evict a resident. (See **Appendix** for eviction rules.)

If you or Medicaid aren't paying the nursing home, it might threaten to transfer Mom to the cheapest, lowest-quality facility available. That's one way nursing homes cut their losses.

But if you can't just take Mom's or Grandpa's cash, how can you protect it? Here are three ways to keep the nursing home from eating your loved one's estate.

Community Spouse Resource Allowance

If the patient is married with a community spouse, then a portion of their assets is already protected, even as they apply for Medicaid. (If the patient is single, this section doesn't apply. Please skip ahead to the next section.)

The **Community Spouse Resource Allowance**, or CSRA, sets what is known as the "protected amount" of assets, updated each year. The federal **spousal impoverishment law** specifies the CSRA, preventing

Medicaid from combining the assets and income of both spouses to pay for care, which would leave the community spouse unable to support themselves. (At this writing in 2022, the CSRA is a maximum of $137,400.)

Medicaid tallies all assets owned by either or both parties in a marriage as of what's called the **snapshot date**—the date either party is admitted to a nursing home. At that time, if one spouse has only $2,500 in savings but the other has $500,000, then Medicaid considers *each* spouse as having access to $502,500. That's the snapshot number. (I use this extremely lopsided example to show how, well, extreme the policy is.)

Fortunately, the CSRA allots that a maximum of $137,400 is protected. Again, this is the maximum amount of the total married couple's assets the community spouse can keep when the other enters a nursing home and has not yet qualified for Medicaid nursing home coverage. Anything above and beyond this number then becomes the focus of your asset protection strategy.

Now, I want to clarify that while $137,400 is the maximum protected amount, it is not the *minimum* protected amount. Let's say you and your spouse have, for simplicity's sake, $137,500 between the two of you. *Great!* you might have been thinking. Do you get to keep all but $100 away from the nursing home?

Well . . . no. The CSRA program has a state-by-state formula that determines the minimum you will be allowed to shield during the Medicaid look-back period. (Please see the **Appendix** for more details on how to calculate the CSRA for your exact situation and state.)

Once you know how much money you have left over, you can use the remaining three strategies described below to protect the rest of the estate.

Irrevocable Funeral Expense Trust

As we covered earlier, nursing homes encourage families to set up funeral expense trusts. Why? 1) They don't want to get stuck with a body. 2) As the adage says, "There's nothing guaranteed in life but death and taxes." A funeral is an inevitable expense.

Yet talking to a salesperson at a funeral home right after moving Grandma into a nursing home is stressful. The salesperson will sell you caskets, prayer cards, and other merchandise. Some families are ready for this, but most don't want the hassle and simply want to protect their assets without deciding on all the details.

I am not advocating that you avoid unpleasant necessities. Whether in the short-, mid-, or long-term, the financial side of funeral planning for your loved one is a *must,* and it can be done quickly and simply. You should set up an **irrevocable funeral expense trust** for a living spouse, too. You need to make sure that the nursing home can't touch their assets. Remember, traditional life insurance policies with cash values over $1,500 count as an asset and must be cashed out and spent down! You cannot keep them. Only irrevocable funeral expense trusts and other specialized instruments are exempt from consideration as an asset.

Even if you understand why you should set up a funeral expense trust, the law requires a licensed professional to be involved. Our organization can set up trusts to protect your assets in as little as one business day. We can do everything electronically, via snail mail, or in person, and we've been at it for over thirty years.

When planning *your* funeral, ask this question: "Do I make my kids pay for it, or should I pay for it now?"

If you have $10,000 or less left, most or all of it will go toward funeral expenses. Unless you prefer direct cremation, which is less expensive.

Each state has its own limit on how much money you can place in a funeral expense trust. In some states like Pennsylvania, individual counties set the limit. These limits are critical, for if you exceed the limits, the trust is no longer exempt and will create a penalty period. (See the **Appendix** for your state's limits.)

Note that you don't want to max out this specific trust unless you actually intend to use it. Don't put in $15,000 if you're planning for a $3,000 cremation; the remaining amount will be returned to the deceased's estate. Once it goes into the estate, it is subject to Medicaid estate recovery. Fund only enough to cover the cost of the funeral for the individual in the nursing home.

Your elder loved one isn't the only one who stands to benefit from specialized irrevocable trusts. Your extended family can be helped by trusts, too, and these trusts can be funded to the maximum. Here's how.

Irrevocable Burial Space Item Trust

Perhaps the most important strategy in this book, an **irrevocable burial space item trust** covers only specific merchandise, not services. Compared to a funeral expense trust, the line items in the contract are more limited. You can allot money to cover a **burial space item** such as a casket, a vault, or an urn in the contract. You can also include one service, which is the opening and closing of graves. In most states, up to $15,000 can be protected in each of these trusts. Unlike the funeral expense trusts, you can create these for lots of different family members.

You don't see irrevocable burial space item trusts as often because few funeral homes or elder care attorneys are trained to set these up, and doing so incorrectly can cause serious issues such as Medicaid penalty periods. Sadly, nursing homes almost never tell their residents' families about irrevocable burial space item trusts, even though **they are the best possible asset protection strategy for most people.**

Every child—and all the children's spouses—of the individual in the nursing home should have an irrevocable burial space item trust. In effect, these are life insurance policies. When the nursing home resident's survivors pass away, their families receive lump sum payments.

Let's take my grandma again. She received $87,000 from the sale of her home to my cousin. Six of her descendants are parking the $87,000 into six individual life insurance policies of $14,000 each. These policies are placed inside an irrevocable burial space item trust. The funds are earmarked for burial space items. When the six descendants pass away, their families will get $14,000 apiece, tax-free.

These are inevitable expenses, anyway. Instead of the money being lost to the nursing home, it will be returned to the family. Grandma is taking care of her kids, grandkids, and even great-grandkids financially because any money not used for burial space items goes tax-free to those family members' estates.

If someone has a lot of children, irrevocable burial space item trusts can often be sufficient to protect all a family's life savings from the nursing home. But what if the nursing home resident has few descendants and a lot of money? This is where the **single premium immediate annuity**, also known as SPIA, becomes relevant.

Single Premium Immediate Annuities

A single premium immediate **annuity**, also called a Medicaid annuity, is the most complicated instrument described yet. There's a heavy fee for this vehicle. You'll pay an elder care attorney and a licensed insurance agent to guide you through the process. There are no commissions on this product, so the agent has to charge a fee, but the costs are well worth it in certain circumstances. Expect total costs of this service to range from $5,000 to $20,000.

If your estate or your loved one's estate is already being eaten, the annuity can protect at least half of the remaining cash value. Let's say a person's estate is worth $215,000. Subtracting attorney and insurance agent fees of $15,000 leaves $200,000. If the person is single, we can protect half of that money, or $100,000. If a husband or wife is still living, all $200,000 can be transferred to that spouse via the annuity; there is no dividing it.

Here's another example that shows the combination of two strategies. A single mother has an estate worth $205,000, but irrevocable burial estate trusts can protect only $25,000. An elder law attorney would transfer half of the remaining $180,000, or $90,000, to her only daughter, triggering a Medicaid penalty period.

The penalty period is a function of the gift amount divided by something called a divisor rate. Let's say your state's divisor rate is $9,000 a month. In our example, $90,000 was transferred to the daughter out of her mom's estate. The penalty period is 90,000 divided by 9,000, or ten months. When the penalty period kicks in, Medicaid says they won't pay for care for ten months.

However, at the same time that the attorney transfers this cash to the daughter, he places the remaining $90,000 in the annuity. The annuity creates an income of $9,000 a month for the mother to pay the nursing home during the penalty period, thereby eliminating the negative impact of the penalty period.

During the five-year look-back period, Medicaid looks for assets, not income. An annuity "converts" assets to income, thereby escaping the look-back period. Medicaid has income caps, so the annuity must be structured carefully so as not to exceed these limits, but there are no income limits before your loved one is on Medicaid or during the penalty period.

Going back to our example: At the end of the penalty period, Mom has no assets and thus can apply for Medicaid. The $90,000 she gifted to her daughter is not considered a recoverable asset. *Medicaid cannot take it.* So the daughter walks away with half of Mom's assets.

When set up properly, a single premium immediate annuity converts a disqualifying asset into qualifying income. This is what elder law attorneys do in crisis planning, which is what they call the period when your loved one is in a nursing home.

An annuity is the ideal vehicle if you're caught off guard by the nursing home eating your estate, and the funeral expense and irrevocable burial space item trusts won't suffice. It's perfect if you're still married. You can protect almost your entire estate because the money won't be divided in half. It also makes sense if you're single or don't have many children or grandchildren, but you have a lot of money. Losing half of your estate isn't ideal, but it's better than losing everything.

In my grandma's case, we're not doing an annuity because there are so many descendants for whom to create the irrevocable burial space item trusts. It doesn't make sense for our situation, but it might make sense for yours.

So, how do you get started?

Do This Next

Contact us at www.nursinghometrusts.org, and we'll create the funeral expense and irrevocable burial space item trusts for you. We do this for free because we do receive a commission, just like an insurance agent.

Or, go to a local funeral home to set up the funeral expense trust. We have relationships with over eight hundred across the country. If you contact us, we'll make sure they do it right.

Family law and estate planning attorneys rarely do single premium immediate annuities. We work with the specialized kind of elder law attorneys you will need.

If you want to do it all yourself, I recommend visiting the website of the National Academy of Elder Law Attorneys (www.NAELA.org) to find a specialized elder law attorney who can set up a single premium immediate annuity. I recommend that you still get in touch with us because you'll need licensed insurance agents with the necessary expertise to purchase the annuity.

Remember Theresa, from Chapter 1? She's the ninety-three-year-old nursing home trusts client who, together with her daughter, was worried sick about a nursing home seizing her money. We gave them a plan that includes everything you've read about in this chapter.

In the end, we managed to protect $85,000 of Theresa's remaining $100,000. That money didn't matter to Rachel and her own family. She was already well off. What made her happiest was that our conversation put her in a position of power and helped her secure victory for Mom. She was proud of herself for not letting her mother get taken like a sucker. In that one conversation, we debunked the big lie and protected a small fortune.

Maybe you assume the best of nursing homes. Perhaps you have long-term care insurance, or you're in the first month of Medicare. Thinking that a big powerful company will do good is naive. Corporations have no feelings. They have profit and loss statements, shareholder distribution and accountability, and stock prices. Your mom (or dad, grandparent, or spouse) is just a source of revenue for them.

Dealing with the nursing home business office involves hours of conversation and signing documents. And they'll never bring up annuities or irrevocable burial space item trusts.

I've visited over seventy nursing homes and talked to business office managers at most of them. They all have had residents who were represented by competent elder care attorneys or www.nursinghometrusts.org. Annuities and irrevocable trusts come across their desks every day. They know about these ways to protect your money, but they won't bring them to your attention.

Even if you find a nursing home with compassionate staff, financial decisions aren't made at the local level. More than 99 percent of nursing homes are owned by corporations with huge portfolios—and they make the financial decisions. The business office manager is just reading a script prepared by the corporate attorneys, complete with weasel clauses. Corporate entities don't care if you protect your life savings, only that they continue to make their money.

This chapter tackled one big lie. Next, we'll expose another big lie: "They'll do right by us."

CHAPTER 3

— • —

IF YOU'VE JUST MOVED INTO LONG-TERM CARE, READ THIS

Author's Note: The content of this chapter is specifically for readers or their loved ones who have recently moved into a nursing home. Medicare may still be covering long-term care expenses—but only for the next several weeks. Soon, the Medicaid spend-down period begins.

I've heard people voice another assumption with complete conviction: "The nursing home will do what's right; they won't take Mom's money if they don't have to."

Hearing this always stuns and saddens me. We want to believe the best of people and the organizations to whom we entrust our loved ones. But there is a harsh lesson that someone whose loved one has been placed in a nursing home needs to learn. If you fit that description, this chapter is for you.

Let me tell you a story. I was sitting in the boardroom at the headquarters of one of the largest nursing home corporations in the United States. A colleague and I were trying to run a pilot program for nursing home residents in a few of their facilities. The two of us wanted to help residents learn about what we talked about in the last chapter.

At first, the CEO bought into the idea. He knew the strategies you could deploy to protect your funds. But in the end, he viewed our program as a disruption to business. Having people coming in and out of nursing care facilities got in the staff's way. He recognized the huge benefit to individuals, but it did not improve the company's bottom line.

"This meant nothing to our revenue," he said. He was right. Even if we'd protected hundreds of millions of dollars of individual funds, it would've meant nothing to the corporation. Nursing homes don't care whether the money comes from private pay or Medicaid, only that it keeps flowing. Protecting estates doesn't improve their cash flow.

We Have a Problem

The vast majority of nursing homes are owned by massive publicly traded companies. So, nursing homes themselves don't make the financial decisions. Their shareholders do—rather, all decisions must be made in the interest of financial value. Many nursing homes have a department called **revenue cycle management** that focuses on managing the transition from private pay to public pay. That happens at the corporate level, reviewed by corporate attorneys.

Although nursing homes don't care whether money comes from private pay or public pay, they are concerned about private money running out before you get onto Medicaid. Nursing homes don't want you to trigger a penalty period during which you are ineligible for Medicaid but your private money is gone. If that happens, they'll start taking losses. Neither they nor their corporate owners want that.

I consult with a cremation services provider out of Cincinnati, Ohio. The founder's grandmother lost $500,000 to a nursing home due to lack of preparation. The grandmother is still alive today, and her whole estate has been taken. Everything is gone.

This was not a poor family. The son of the woman in the nursing home is a man of means who runs several medical offices in North Carolina. Because their family had a high net worth, they weren't concerned until it was too late. He was not angry until he realized this didn't need to happen.

All nursing home horror stories end the same—families who trust the nursing home to "do the right thing" lose everything to them. We talk to folks who say, "I had half a million when Dad went into the nursing home, and it's gone now. What can we do to get it back?"

"It's too late," I tell them. "Once the money is gone, it's gone. You're never going to see that money again."

In fact, I know a guy who sells data to senior living companies looking to build new assisted living facilities, memory care units, and nursing homes. One of the most important data points the decision-makers look at when deciding where to build is the average estate value of homeowners and individuals living in that zip code. Why? Because they know that in most cases, the senior living company can capture all of that estate. Most families don't plan effectively; they know this. To the publicly traded corporation, it's only a matter of time before your loved one's financial legacy is theirs. Your chance to question any information the nursing home gives is when the nursing home brings it up. After that, it's too late.

Families who realize that the nursing home will take their loved one's entire life savings often try to solve that problem by distributing the money around the family. Big mistake. It's a do-it-yourself tactic that triggers the Medicaid penalty period you learned about in Chapter 1. The formula dictates a delay in Medicaid payments kicking in based on the amount of money that was transferred.

This leads to the worst-case scenario: Mom or Dad's money is gone, but Medicaid won't pay the nursing home. Sure, the nursing home might have to take you to court to try and get the money back (maybe you'll even win), but in the meantime ,they will move your loved one to the cheapest available facility, where there's a higher risk of elder abuse and other such horrors. In the most extreme situations, they will evict.

Most nursing home staff don't know about the methods you can use to protect your legacy. Only the business office knows about instruments such as irrevocable burial space item trusts or single premium immediate annuities. Even then, their job is not to protect your family—it's to protect the nursing home's profits.

I know of only one nursing home that informed their residents of these strategies, and it wasn't even their official policy. The business office manager was a sharp woman with a strong sense of ethics. When dealing with potential clients, she gave the usual spiel to sell the benefits of the home, determined their financial situation, found out how long they would pay privately, then pinpointed when they would apply for Medicaid. After that, she would say, "You need to talk to this elder care attorney in town."

The attorney would visit the nursing home three or four times a week to talk to residents and help them understand what would happen to their finances. The business manager would send clients his way.

This situation benefited everybody. The patients received skilled care, their families received professional help with their finances, and the attorney and the nursing home enjoyed a steady stream of business. All it took was some extra effort from the business office manager. As far as I know, there was nothing in it for her. She did it because it was the right thing to do.

Odds are, you won't find an ethical nursing home that helps you protect your finances. It's up to you to look after your family. Let's talk about how.

What to Do about It

As stated at the outset, this chapter was written for patients and their families who are new to nursing homes. If you or your loved one is undergoing nursing home rehabilitation, recovery and return to normal life is expected. It may not make sense for you to sell the home or take other drastic measures like we discussed in Chapter 2. On the other hand, if you expect the patient needs long-term care, you need to take extra steps.

In Chapter 1, we covered the types of trusts and annuities you can use to protect your estate. In this section, we'll explore how to use these instruments for your specific situation.

The first thing you should ask is whether the patient will be undergoing short-term rehab, or if the move to the nursing home will be permanent. The answer will determine your next course of action.

Don't think you can afford to wait. The unexpected can and will happen. Sad to say, many people think Grandma will just be going to the nursing home for rehab, and Medicare will cover it all. But she doesn't improve. Then she develops an infection. As the days pass, Grandma's condition worsens—and Medicare stops payments.

Medicare is for rehabilitation and improvement. Once the patient stops showing improvement, or after one hundred days of care, Medicare stops paying. That's when you start pulling out your private money.

You can't assume that once Grandma is in long-term care, you can take your time doing research. By the time you've spent weeks doing that, you're already spent thousands of dollars. So it's all about educating yourself ASAP. Once it's determined whether the patient will be on long-term care or short-term rehab, you need to act.

Let's take a deep dive into some options we touched on in Chapter 2.

Gifting Your Home

Your home is your most valuable asset. Protecting it should be a priority. As discussed in Chapter 2, there are two main ways to do this.

If your loved one is married with a community spouse—a spouse who lives in the community and is not in a nursing home or on Medicaid—then when the patient enters the nursing home, the spouse gets to keep the family home, even after their loved one dies. That is the most straightforward case.

If the patient is single or widowed, then you need to proceed with caution. Simply gifting the home to someone would trigger a Medicaid penalty period. However, there are three scenarios that allow you to freely gift a home without penalty.

The first is for the patient to give away the house to a child under twenty-one years old, a child who is blind, or a child who is permanently disabled.

The second is for the patient to gift the home to an adult child who lived in the home and provided care to their parent for a minimum of two years prior to entering the nursing home.

The third is for the patient to gift the home to a sibling, as long as the sibling has ownership of an equity interest in the home and has lived in it for at least a year prior to the patient's admission to the nursing home. Deeding even 1 percent of the ownership of the home to the sibling would be enough, as long as the sibling paid market price. A year later, the patient can enter the nursing home and safely transfer to the home completely to the sibling.

If these scenarios don't apply to you, there's still the option of selling the home to a family member at a reasonable market price. Selling it at $1 counts as a gift. To attain a reasonable market price, either hire a professional appraiser, or multiply the assessed tax value by the **common level ratio**.

You can find more information about this in Chapter 2.

Irrevocable Funeral Expense Trust

As we covered in the previous chapter, an irrevocable funeral expense trust is a way to prefund the funeral while you or your loved one is still alive. This is often the only method a nursing home will disclose to you, because they don't want to cover the cost of the burial.

Whether you're going home after rehab to live another fifteen years, or you'll be living in a nursing home for the rest of your life, it makes sense to get an irrevocable funeral expense trust. This will ease the burden on your family when the inevitable happens and keep the nursing home from touching your funds.

Put only enough money into these trusts to cover your actual funeral expenses with a modest margin for inflation, however. That could be $3,000 for a simple cremation or $15,000 for a traditional funeral. After paying for funeral expenses, any remaining monies in this trust will be returned to the deceased's estate, which Medicaid can seize. That's why we don't overfund these trusts.

If the individual facing nursing home care has a spouse, always set up an additional trust for them as well. Remember, in a nursing home situation, you will "use it or lose it."

Irrevocable Burial Space Item Trust

On paper, this vehicle covers burial goods such as caskets, vaults, and urns. It cannot be used to cover services, except for opening and closing the grave. In practice, it's a life insurance policy stuffed inside a specialized trust. Once the individual covered by the trust passes away, his family receives a tax-free lump-sum payment.

Let's go back to the example of Grandma developing an infection and Medicare ceasing payments. Overnight, you've gone from Medicare paying for everything to owing $10,000 a month. You have to pay $300 a day just for nursing home expenses.

If the patient has kids, and the kids have spouses of their own, set up this trust for everyone right now. It doesn't cost anything to set it up. You cannot afford to wait. Every day you delay is $300 gone from your family's estate. While there is a cap on how much money you can lock away in an irrevocable burial space item trust, at least you've protected *some* money for the long term.

Single Premium Immediate Annuities

This complicated instrument, also called a Medicaid annuity, requires an elder care attorney and a licensed insurance agent. After covering attorney and agent fees, the annuity will protect half of the patient's estate—or all of it if the patient has a living spouse.

While expensive (costing approximately $7,500 to $20,000), this is the best financial protection for someone with a lot of money but few family members. If that's you, then set up an annuity now, *before* the patient goes into a nursing home.

The idea is to use the annuity to transform disqualifying assets into qualifying income. In the case of a nursing home resident with a community spouse, everything (minus fees) can be protected. For a single individual we use the "half-a-loaf" strategy, which purposefully triggers a Medicaid penalty period by gifting half of the money to a person of choice while simultaneously creating an income stream via the annuity to cover the penalty period. After the annuity expires, the family member keeps the money while the patient applies for Medicaid. Complicated, I know, but that's why these are always done with licensed supervision.

There's no need to do this if you're expecting short-term rehab. However, if the patient is expected to move into long-term care, the annuity makes sense. It takes a while to set up. You cannot afford to wait until the last minute. Once you're certain the patient will be going into long-term care—*not* rehab—get the ball rolling.

Accounting of Assets

Whether your loved one is facing a long-term or permanent stay in a nursing home, you'll need an accounting of all assets up to and including the last five years of transactions. These assets include a house or other real estate, any vehicles, insurance policies, retirement accounts such as 401(k)s and IRAs, and long-term care insurance.

The purpose of this five-year look-back period is to find any transactions that might trigger a Medicaid penalty period. For example, if your loved one gifted $50,000 to a son or daughter, that could create a penalty period.

You or an attorney will need to account for the assets. Should you choose to hire a lawyer, you should look for an elder law attorney who understands the nuances of these situations. Before hiring an elder law attorney, contact us for help at www.nursinghometrusts.org. Otherwise, go to www.NAELA.org, which provides a searchable database of accredited elder law attorneys.

Most attorneys charge $7,500 to $20,000 for the full package. This includes:

- A full accounting of resources, including the last five years' worth of transactions;

- Determining which financial strategies to deploy, likely including the irrevocable funeral expense trust, irrevocable burial space item trust, and the Medicaid annuity (their favorite);
- Completing the Medicaid application.

The high fees involved in this approach often don't make sense to someone with less than $100,000 in assets. If that's you, put everything into irrevocable burial space item trusts and irrevocable funeral expense trusts to avoid fees.

For someone with assets worth $150,000 or more, the fees start to make clear sense. Spending $20,000 to protect $130,000 out of $150,000 is a no-brainer. Even then, the entire estate could be protected using irrevocable funeral expense and burial space item trusts for large families with many children and spouses. However, hiring a specialized attorney can also make sense if you have a small family and assets of about $500,000 or more.

While hiring an attorney will cost you more, it also might help you protect a bigger share of your assets. Although attorneys offer bundled services, an attorney will need a licensed insurance agent to deploy most of the financial products in their arsenal. So contact us; we can take care of that without having to bring in an inexperienced third party.

The best elder care attorney I know has a team of twelve under him. One person vets bank account records; another goes through all real estate investments, 401(k)s, and so on. While his operation runs like a machine, processing a case could take weeks, even a few months.

The time commitment involved in working with a lawyer is a function of the family's willingness to provide information. Just hiring an attorney doesn't give the legal team access to Grandma's bank accounts. You need to produce the information when your lawyer needs it to avoid delays.

But if funeral expense trusts and burial space item trusts will be enough to protect your family's assets, www.nursinghometrusts.org can set them up for you.

Let's say Grandma has $80,000 in cash. She no longer has a house or a car, but she has a life insurance policy that needs to be liquidated. Grandma was on assisted living, and two weeks from now, she'll be transferred to a nursing home for long-term care. After two weeks, you'll start paying $300 a day.

If you engage us, we will carry out a detailed analysis of your situation and draw up trusts sufficient to protect Grandma's assets. Everything can be signed digitally and completed within forty-eight hours. It's the fastest solution available.

If you don't have an attorney, or if your attorney doesn't handle Medicaid applications, the nursing home's business office will. We can give them a packet that documents the trusts we've established for your family. The business office will use that information to complete the Medicaid application. It puts the onus on them to do it right, because they won't get paid if they do it wrong.

Now here's the number-one thing you can do to keep you and your loved one from getting taken advantage of . . .

Respect the Transition

This is a transition period. Your parents cared for you during your entire early childhood, teenage years, and even young adulthood. Now it's time for you to care for them.

I am the father of three children. My role as their caretaker is one I can't neglect. And when the roles reverse, I don't want my kids to neglect me. Because the nursing home, the lawyers, the doctors, and the physical therapists won't advocate for me in the way my children can.

It's your role to find the professionals who will take care of Mom or Dad. Do it now so you can get back to focusing on your loved one, not stressing about finances. The last thing you want is to get stuck thinking, *If only I'd done this . . .*

You want to be able to bring the kids in for stories and chicken soup with Mom. To look through old family photos and relive memories. You want to be present in the moment, not fretting over that $300 per day while taking the kids to see Dad for what will be the last time.

It's impossible to focus on life's most important moments when there's a sword hanging over your family's financial legacy. You want to unload all that baggage before your loved one even enters the nursing home. Act now, save yourself all the stress, and advocate for those who took care of you as a child.

CHAPTER 4

———————— • ————————

IF YOU MIGHT NEED A NURSING HOME IN THE NEXT FIVE YEARS, READ THIS

Author's Note: The content of this chapter is specifically for readers or their loved ones who expect to need long-term care within the next five years. Five years is the Medicaid look-back period that may result in penalties down the line if unwise financial decisions are made. This chapter shows how to avoid them.

I f you or your loved one might need a nursing home within five years, this chapter is for you. Maybe you're not sure you need it, but you see the warning signs. Perhaps Dad's not getting around like he used to. Maybe Mom's forgetting things that she never would have a few years ago. Whatever the case may be, you are contemplating a move to a nursing home.

That may mean all the kids get their inheritance early, perhaps $50,000 to $100,000 each. Somebody will get Mom's house. You'll also want to protect her nest egg while she is downsizing.

You might think it's simple, but when cases like these go wrong, they get ugly. The worst even involve attorneys, and not the kind who help you plan in advance.

I talked to a guy named John in a situation just like this. His mom was on an even keel. She lived off Social Security and had no major expenses. Her real asset was her home. The family had built the house generations ago. It was worth half a million dollars, and she sold it to her son for just $50,000.

One day, John's mom broke her hip. She went to the hospital and later to a nursing home. Her condition wasn't improving, so she had to transition to long-term care. She had only $15,000 in cash and was ready to apply for Medicaid.

Now, within the five-year look-back period, you have to sell a home at fair market value to avoid a penalty period. In most states, the fair market value is determined by an appraisal. In some states you can also base the fair market value off tax assessments multiplied by the common level ratio. (See the **Appendix**.) Selling a home below that price is treated as a gift to the new owner and triggers a penalty period.

Naturally, Medicaid examined the home sale. They discovered that when Mom sold the family home to John, she created a delta of $450,000: the home's actual value of $500,000 minus the actual purchase price of $50,000. As a result, Medicaid considered the home sale a gift. That triggered a penalty period.

The penalty period is calculated by dividing the gifted amount by the daily **penalty divisor**, which is the average daily cost of nursing home care. This value varies from state to state. In Pennsylvania as of 2022, the daily penalty divisor is $482.50. Here, 450,000 divided by 482.50 amounts to a penalty period of 932 days—over *two and a half years*!

Mom had only $15,000 in cash left. The nursing home was at risk of not getting paid, and Medicaid wouldn't pay for nursing home care for 932 days! John's family had to come up with $450,000 to cover the nursing home bills. John thought his only option was to sell the family home.

That kind of mess is all too common, and it's almost impossible to untangle. The family home is the average American's only real asset. Most people don't have $450,000 in stocks or other liquid assets. If John's mom had given away $450,000 in cash (not assets) within the five-year look-back period, that still would have created a penalty period.

Maybe you think there's plenty of time to sort out your family estate. You believe you can gift the inheritance early, so everything will be OK. Plus, Mom still exercises daily but is ready to move into a small apartment or a condo. You don't foresee a need for a nursing home.

But then an emergency like COVID-19, stage 2 cancer, or dementia strikes. All the independent years you thought Mom had left are stripped away. Now every transaction that happened in the past five years is under scrutiny.

Maybe Mom sold her gold coin collection to your older brother for 10 percent of its actual value. That 90 percent difference in value will be flagged if the gift occurred during the five-year look-back period. That—along with any other gifts she made during that time—will trigger a penalty period.

So stay on your toes. Be ready to act. Here's how.

How to Protect the Family Estate During Medicaid's Look-Back Period

Perhaps Dad has fewer years of independent living left than you thought. Or maybe he has five to ten years but is living alone at seventy-two. Either way, *do not* distribute gifts from the estate. If it's possible you could need a nursing home in the next five years, you need to view everything you do through the lens of the five-year look-back period. Medicaid will look at any money leaving Dad's account that he wouldn't spend normally.

Expenditures such as repairing the roof or buying a new lawn mower are considered reasonable. He can spend $25,000 making the bathroom handicapped accessible without a problem. It's when Dad starts transferring money to other people and not getting equal value in return that issues arise. If Dad claims he spent $25,000 on a kitchen sink, Medicaid will scrutinize the transaction because it's not reasonable.

Incoming money will also be examined. If $15,000 just appears in Mom's account, it will raise a red flag. Medicaid will ask how she got that money. Did she sell an asset for below the fair market value? If so, it will be considered a gift.

The rule of thumb is that Medicaid scrutinizes transactions of $500 or more. Let's say Mom writes her kids $200 checks on their birthdays. They won't be flagged if there's a consistent pattern over several years. But if she gave you $10,000 three months ago, that's a different story.

You need to be aware of every single transaction the patient made in the five years prior to a hypothetical nursing home admission. Because every high-value transaction will be scrutinized, and every one of them could create a penalty period. All those little penalty periods can stack up into a huge one. You don't want to be taken by surprise!

If a lot of money has been gifted out of the estate and Dad is entering a nursing home much sooner than planned, talk to an elder law attorney immediately.

Otherwise, you can create a nightmare scenario if you spend from the estate. The nursing home might threaten to move Mom to a terrible place in the middle of nowhere. Or you might be forced to pay for care. At that point, you're beyond my help.

To keep the family home, consider the "adult child caregiver" scenario. If Mom has a grown child who's willing to provide live-in care for at least two years before the Medicaid application, the child gets to keep her home.

Now, this is specific care to support her daily activities and routine—cooking, cleaning, help with bathing, and so on. No medical care is required. The government views your taking care of your parent for two years or more as offsetting two years of Medicaid bills. So they allow you to keep the home.

Another scenario that affords easy protection of the home is if the individual needing nursing home care has a child under twenty-one or a permanently disabled child of any age. Developmental disabilities and physical disabilities both count. That person needs to live in the family home with the parent. This exempts transfers of the home to children who meet these standards from the Medicaid look-back. So Mom or Dad can gift that individual the home without negative consequences.

A third method is holding assets in a kind of informal **escrow**. This requires entrusting a family member with the money for five years so that ultimately, it is no longer considered an asset after five years. This approach requires that you have a trusted, responsible family member available.

Let's say Mom has $250,000, or a house worth the same amount. She could give that $250,000 or house to a trusted family member, who would safeguard it and not spend it. If Mom doesn't require a nursing home for five years, you get to keep the $250,000 or the house free and clear. But if Mom has to go into a nursing home within those five years, the trusted family member must transfer the assets back to Mom. We can then use the other strategies discussed in earlier chapters to protect the assets, and no penalty period will be triggered.

The next strategy is ideal for families with more significant wealth. Imagine something happens next week that puts you in a nursing home. Nursing homes near you charge $100,000 a year. And you have $2 million in cash.

First things first. Carve out $500,000 of that $2 million estate to cover five years of hypothetical nursing home care. Give away or donate everything else to whomever you want. This gives you a cushion for five years while protecting the rest of the estate. When you apply for Medicaid five years from now, the $1.5 million of assets you gave away will be outside the look-back period. If you happen to need a nursing home immediately, you have $500,000 to cover your expenses for five years till the penalty period elapses from the transfer of the $1.5 million.

Alternatively, or perhaps concurrently, you could also consider setting aside money to buy long-term care insurance. Let's say the premium costs $10,000. You can take that money out of your $2 million estate, maybe in addition to the $500,000 you're setting aside, and use it to pay for five years of long-term care insurance.

Ensure that the long-term care policy will pay benefits for the full five years—some policies cover only a shorter period. That way, if you suddenly need a nursing home, the long-term care policy will cover you during the five-year look-back period. By spending $10,000 on long-term care premiums, you could in theory protect as much money as you want without any legal restrictions.

Another possibility is a hybrid long-term care policy. This product contains a death benefit. Payments for long-term care reduces the death benefit; whatever is not spent will be passed on to the family. The best-case scenario is never having to use the policy at all. For example, let's say a person with a hybrid policy dies suddenly without using it to pay for nursing home expenses. The entire death benefit will be passed on to the family.

This strategy applies to families with a higher net worth and those who are sure they're more than five years away from using a nursing home. We'll discuss it more in the next chapter. For now, let's take a look at some financial vehicles to safeguard your estate.

Financial Vehicles to Keep Your Money in the Family

In addition to the strategies covered above, we can also use three financial vehicles to protect your estate. These are the irrevocable funeral expense trust, the irrevocable burial space item trust, and the single premium immediate annuity. We covered them in greater detail in Chapter 2. In this section, we will explore how you can use them to fit your current situation.

Irrevocable Funeral Expense Trust

An irrevocable funeral expense trust prefunds a funeral by locking up money for this purpose. You definitely should set one up because it's an inevitable cost. Even if you live for another twenty years, you will need it eventually.

If you do end up in a nursing home, this money is secured. The nursing home can't touch it. This is the one method the nursing home will tell you about to protect your estate, because they don't want to pay for a funeral.

However, you need to fund the trust accurately. Park only enough money to cover your expected funeral costs. If you're planning for a $3,000 cremation but fund the trust with $10,000, the remaining $7,000 will return to the deceased's estate after the funeral. At that point, Medicaid will come for it.

Irrevocable Burial Space Item Trust

An irrevocable burial space item trust covers merchandise, such as caskets or urns. Services such as a limousine, driving, or funeral direction should not be included in these trusts.

Set up irrevocable burial space item trusts for the family members of the patient. All children and children's spouses can have one of these established. In most states, the limit is $15,000. When the family member passes away, the next-of-kin receive the funds in these trusts. Any funds left over after covering burial space merchandise can be kept tax-free.

The trust must cover *only* items—the only allowable service is the opening and closing of the grave. If the irrevocable burial space item trust covers other services, it's no longer an exempted asset.

Single Premium Immediate Annuity

If you do nothing else this chapter says to protect your assets, and at some time in the future end up in a nursing home with significant assets in your name, you'll still be able to use the single premium immediate annuity. If you're paying the nursing home now and thinking about applying for Medicaid, the single premium immediate annuity is definitely for you. If you can't relate to either scenario, you don't need to worry about single premium immediate annuities.

Please also note that these specialized annuities are for crisis planning situations only. It's not something an elder care attorney would sell to you or recommend if you aren't applying for Medicaid immediately. This annuity can convert disqualifying assets into qualifying income, but if you use it several years in advance, the annuity payments would become assets again, and thereby count against you in a Medicaid application, undermining the entire purpose. Single premium immediate annuities need to be timed alongside the Medicaid application for maximum effect. When used this way, and this way alone, they are extremely effective tools for nursing home asset protection.

Other Strategies to Consider

Maybe neither you nor your loved one will need a nursing home within five years. But you must be ready if that timetable shortens. If you have more flexibility now, there are other strategies you can use. For instance, you can deploy long-term care policies with a whole life element. These complicated products are almost always sold in the context of working with an elder care attorney. Contact us at www.nursinghometrusts.org, or speak to an elder care attorney to find out more.

Wealthy families can explore **irrevocable estate planning trusts** or dynasty trusts. Let's say you have $1 million in cash or investments. You could set up an irrevocable estate planning trust and place the money in an insurance product within it. Even if the market tanks, you won't lose any money. The trust owns all the funds, and no one can remove them.

A lawyer can customize the trust to suit your situation. The product we sell—an insurance-funded, irrevocable estate planning trust—lets you set aside as much money as you want in the trust. After five years, no one can touch the funds. When you die, the trust will pay out the death benefit tax-free to whomever you like. This is a free and simple solution for someone who wants to leave the kids a few hundred thousand dollars. These prefab trusts are a great solution for most families that don't have the assets or complicated estates that would justify a costly, custom trust an attorney has built for their unique situation. We will cover the irrevocable estate planning trust in greater detail in Chapter 5.

Getting back to John, his story often ends with the nursing home intimidating the family into coughing up $450,000. In most situations, that means selling the home.

If the penalty period runs to three to four years and covers hundreds of thousands of dollars, lawyer up. There's a chance the nursing home will settle. A good attorney can negotiate them down to $200,000 and have them cover Mom for the penalty period.

Even if you have several years before a nursing home situation arises, you must get an irrevocable funeral expense trust right away. We can set one up for you in fifteen minutes with an e-signature. I invite you to contact us right away at www.nursinghometrusts.org. We'll listen to your situation and set up every applicable measure to protect your finances.

Suppose you're sure that a nursing home event is definitely five or more years out, possibly ten years or more. Mom is fifty-nine, Dad is sixty-two, and there is no family history of heart attacks or Alzheimer's. But you are a new parent thinking about your own legacy. Your parents may also be thinking of their grandchildren. If this situation describes your family, the next chapter is for you.

CHAPTER 5

———— • ————

IF YOU'RE MORE THAN FIVE YEARS AWAY FROM ASSISTED LIVING, READ THIS

Author's Note: The content of this chapter is specifically for readers or their loved ones who do not anticipate needing a nursing home for at least five to ten years. This is the most enviable position to be in regarding long-term care relative to those covered in previous chapters.

Whether you skipped to this chapter or you've read the whole book so far, you're among an exclusive few. Most people don't look this far ahead. You're ready to be honest with yourself about what life could look like in ten to fifteen years, and you might be nervous that you're not as prepared as you'd like to be.

I've talked to people who thought they were a decade or two away from long-term care, only to end up there four years later. That assumption cost them hundreds of thousands of dollars and cost their children their legacy.

Whether you have more than you need saved up for your golden years, or you have just a little left over for the kids, it's good to think about this now. You're for whom I'm writing.

This chapter covers using trusts to protect your estate. Trust documents can range in cost from $0 to $20,000 to establish. If you have hundreds of thousands or even millions of dollars in your estate, that modest expense is a no-brainer.

Don't plan in crisis mode. Let me show you how to safeguard your future.

How to Use Trusts

If you're confident that you have at least five years before going into a nursing home, my best advice is to give away everything you don't intend to spend in your lifetime: homes, cars, the millions in your accounts. Get it all out of your name.

It doesn't matter to whom you give your property. It could be family, friends, or charity. As long as it's a permanent transfer and you do it five or more years before a nursing home event, it won't cause any issues with Medicaid. That's because none of those transactions will fall within the five-year look-back period.

What if you don't want to give your wealth away?

Instead of giving money to people, give the money to a trust. A trust is a legal entity, and you can have more than one. For example, one trust can hold your home, and another can hold your other assets.

Trusts can take myriad forms. In this chapter, we will explore six kinds of trusts, from the simplest to the most complicated.

Irrevocable Funeral Expense Trust

An irrevocable funeral expense trust prefunds your funeral. Everyone is going to die, so everyone should have one, whether they have other trusts or not. If you secure the trust early, you can lock in preferential prices as well.

The money parked in the irrevocable funeral expense trust cannot be touched by a nursing home. However, after the funeral, any remaining monies will return to the estate, where they are subject to asset seizure rules. Therefore, fund the trust only enough to cover funeral costs.

For more information on this trust, refer to Chapter 2.

Irrevocable Burial Space Item Trust

An irrevocable burial space item trust covers the cost of goods that go into a burial, such as a casket, a vault, or an urn. This trust is limited to merchandise. Any services listed on the contract besides the opening and the closing of the grave will cause issues with Medicaid.

You should also get this trust for your kids, grandkids, and their spouses. In effect, it's a life insurance policy. After the person covered by the trust passes away, the money goes to the family tax-free and is exempt from Medicaid estate recovery rules. Any money that's left after purchasing the goods is theirs to keep.

Bear in mind that there's a hard limit on the amount you can park in an irrevocable burial space item trust. This limit varies from state to state. If you have a small family, this type of trust may not be enough to protect your entire estate.

As with the previous trust, flip back to Chapter 2 for more information.

Irrevocable Estate Planning Trust

The irrevocable estate planning trust is a no-brainer when you know with great certainty that you're at least five years away from using a nursing home.

If you have money above and beyond what can be protected in the irrevocable funeral and burial space items trusts and want to pass it on tax-free to someone else, this is for you. The money doesn't have to be for your children. You could give it your grandchildren or to charity. In fact, you can list as many beneficiaries as you like and control how much goes to each. These trusts are perfect if you know you're not going to need the money anymore; you just want to keep it from being taken. It's a great way to give a gift without being subjected to the Medicaid look-back period, either.

The money has to sit inside the trust for at least five years before the nursing home event in order not to be considered an asset by Medicaid. After that, it cannot be touched by the nursing home—or anyone, for that matter. The funds in the trust are immediately protected from creditors, lawyers, and probate court. Why? Because it's irrevocable, meaning permanent. The monies can be paid out tax-free only to the beneficiaries named in the trust after you die. So be sure you will never need the money that you place in this trust.

The irrevocable estate planning trust isn't for the uber-wealthy, either. In most cases, the trust has a $2,500 minimum and a $100,000 maximum. We've been able to get carriers to waive that maximum for select clients. Contact us at www.nursinghometrusts.org to find out more.

Irrevocable Income Only Trust

The **irrevocable income only trust** is for people who want their assets out of their name but still want those assets to work for them. Once you put your assets into this trust, you can never get them back. However, you are entitled to the income generated from the assets in the trust.

Imagine you have a portfolio of stocks or real estate, or a business worth $1 million dollars. Your investments pay you $100,000 of dividends or income each year. By locking up your assets in an irrevocable income only trust, you can't take out the principal. But neither can the nursing home after these assets have been in the trust for five years. However, you can receive the income from those assets for the rest of your life.

You'll want to shut that income faucet off once you go into the nursing home so you can apply for Medicaid. The trust itself can state that when a nursing home situation arises, they will give your assets to your children or another designated person or entity.

The irrevocable income only trust is appropriate for a lot of people. It is almost always done in cooperation with an elder law attorney. We can help you find the right attorney to help you set up this trust.

Special Needs Trust

The **special needs trust**, also called a third-party trust or a supplemental needs trust, has a specific scope. It can pay out to a beneficiary only for covering supplemental needs. That does not cover nursing home expenses, but it can pay for many others.

If it's not covered by Medicaid, chances are the special needs trust can cover it. These costs include nonfood groceries, alternative medical therapies, dental work, massages, haircuts, over-the-counter medicines, transportation, furniture, clothing, cell phones, vacations, entertainment, and even attorney fees.

Medicaid will not consider a special needs trust an asset because it's limited to paying only for those supplemental needs. So any money within this trust will not affect your Medicaid application.

Customized Trust

You can hire a lawyer to create a customized trust, depending on how complicated your financial situation is.

Let's say you own a business, land, or multiple homes. You might want the trust's proceeds to go to a complex hierarchy of family members, or you might want to place certain assets in the trust. It will be worth your while to hire an attorney to structure a customized trust for your family and lock down your assets.

However, if your financial situation is simpler, you have fewer assets, and you just want to protect some money for your kids, contact us. If you do need an attorney, we'll work with you directly. Contact us at www. nursinghometrusts.org.

Insurance Tools to Protect Your Estate

Let's look at what else might be available to you, depending on your situation.

Long-Term Care Insurance

A long-term care insurance policy covers nursing home care, home health care, and personal or adult day care. Long-term care policies range from $2,000 to $10,000 per year. Premiums depend on age, health, marital status, and other factors, which is why that range is so broad.

Whatever you might pay for long-term care insurance, there are superior alternatives to it. I recommend instead that you consider many of the alternatives, such as trusts, covered throughout this book. If you set up a good trust with an attorney or through www.nursinghometrusts.org, you won't have to pay nursing home fees. Once you reach a nursing home situation, you'll be on Medicaid.

Here's a hypothetical: Grandma establishes an irrevocable estate trust for her home and $500,000. Even though the money and the home are in the trust, she still lives in the house. The trust pays for repairs and maintenance. She uses her Social Security checks to continue living life as she always has.

Grandma didn't plan on spending that $500,000. It sits there and grows or is preserved. Seven years from now, Grandma breaks a hip, goes into the nursing home, and enrolls in Medicaid. She spends the next three years in the nursing home and passes away. The family now inherits the home and half a million dollars.

That situation was set up for success. We knew Grandma wouldn't need that $500,000. She had Medicare for all her health insurance needs. By using the irrevocable estate trust, she passed on her estate to her family.

Let's look at another scenario. Grandma spends $5,000 a year on long-term care insurance. She lives for seven years before going into the nursing home. That's $35,000 in premiums. If she lives for another three years, the policy payout covers only half of the nursing home fees. She has to spend another $150,000 to cover the rest of her stay.

That's a total expenditure of $185,000. And now there's only $315,000 left for the family. If she lives seven years in the nursing home, the entire estate will be gone.

See why I said there are better options than long-term care? Of course, for people in certain situations, long-term care insurance might make sense.

In Chapters 4 and 5, we discussed people who were on the fence about whether they'd need a nursing home soon. Long-term care insurance is for people in this situation.

Someone deploying this strategy can gift away their entire estate, which normally would subject them to a penalty period if they needed nursing home care within five years. However, in this case, it's a smart move because they've simultaneously purchased a long-term care policy to cover them for a full five years.

Here's how this works. After giving away a ton of money, you buy long-term care insurance covering five years in case you need a nursing home. The premium costs $10,000, and you have $120,000 in your estate. You can give away $110,000 to your kids through an irrevocable trust. Then you take the remaining $10,000 to pay for five years of long-term care insurance.

Should you need a nursing home, you have a long-term care policy to cover you for the five-year look-back period. Otherwise, you'll have to get the money from your family. It's critical to make sure the long-term care policy you buy will pay benefits for a full five years should you need it. Some policies stop paying after shorter periods of care.

This strategy also works for people who don't think a nursing home is a real possibility but are planning their estate. By spending $10,000 on long-term care premiums, you could hypothetically protect an unlimited amount of money.

Should you find yourself in this position, you could also consider a hybrid long-term care policy. This product builds a whole life cash value that can be passed on after death. Suppose you have a family member who pays for a hybrid policy for ten years, then passes away from a heart attack. He never needed nursing home care. The death benefit is passed on to his family.

Long-term care insurance is a highly specialized product that may not be for everyone. If you need help figuring out if you need it, reach out to us.

We'll Help You

Depending on your scenario, my personal advice to you may be different. Most people have $20,000 to $100,000 that they might want to pass on to their children or grandchildren. They don't want it lost to nursing homes or taxes.

We'll help you no matter your situation. For example, we can set up irrevocable estate planning trusts, funeral expense trusts, or burial space item trusts through www.nursinghometrusts.org. It's free, simple, and takes only two days.

CHAPTER 6

———————— • ————————

HOW TO PREVENT THE WORST-CASE SCENARIO

W hen I was in college, the worst happened to my maternal grand-mother, Ruthanne. She was a good grandma—not that there are bad ones. What makes the details I'm about to share with you ironic is the fact that her late husband, Cliff, had owned a funeral home. After his death, Grandma Ruthanne lived alone for ten years. She was in great health and had family in the area. Then all of a sudden, she was diagnosed with leukemia.

Grandma didn't want anyone, including her four kids and grandchil-dren, to see her vulnerable. I didn't know until after she'd passed away that she had dyed her hair red since her late forties. Any of us would have been glad to pay for in-home care, but she wanted to move from Pennsyl-vania to Virginia to live near her sister.

The treatments didn't work, and her cancer progressed. The nursing home burned through her remaining savings; she had nothing left. In the room right next to my grandmother's was the father of a lawyer. He had found a way to protect everything for his family. In the exact same facil-ity, under the exact same care, we lost it all and they protected everything.

At the time, we knew nothing, not even basics such as a funeral expense trust. We didn't have anyone with power of attorney. My grandmother wanted to handle everything herself because she was lucid and coherent until the medications took that from her at the end.

This was the first time I became keyed into the world of nursing home expenses and legacy protection. It would have been possible to protect our estate, but we did nothing.

We learned a hard lesson. You can imagine how differently we are handling my paternal grandmother's final expenses. As of this writing, her house is already safe with my cousin. (See Chapter 2.) We're protecting $87,000 through irrevocable burial space item trusts. The state will have nurses provide her care in her own home, where she has lived her entire life. It's a big difference.

These two anecdotes demonstrate the fates that could befall you if you don't act and the ideal outcome if you do. Even if you feel like it's too late to keep a nursing home from burning through your loved one's assets, it may be possible to protect the rest of the estate.

The irony is that my mother's side of the family has lots of bankers, investors, and entrepreneurs. Grandma Ruthanne's son-in-law was president of a publicly traded New York bank that handled funds for the US Treasury's Troubled Assets Relief Program. Yet in her last years, my grandmother suffered the worst financial fate there could be. Everything she had was taken from her when she was least able to protect it.

On the other hand, my dad's side of the family came from humble roots. They didn't have much wealth or many college degrees. Yet with the information I've gained over the years, the same information you're reading in this book, we're going to take care of my dad's mom. You can take care of your own family, too.

It's not about education, background, or careers. It's about specific, hidden knowledge.

Remember, this is a $300-a-day problem on average. That's $9,000 per month, if not more, depending on your state and city. There is no advantage to waiting. The more time you have, the more options there are.

At Nursing Home Trusts, we hear from people all the time who have lost everything, and we can't help you get it back. Once the nursing home has your assets, they're gone. As time runs out, options decrease. And if you haven't acted, one day there will be no options left. That's why it's vital to reach out to us while we can still protect you.

If a $9,000-a-month inevitable expense, plus the possibility of losing the family home, doesn't motivate you to act, this book isn't for you. It's for people who want to know what's going to happen to Mom's or Dad's estate after they die.

I encourage people to *decide* what will happen, rather than leave it up to the for-profit nursing home. For those who want relief, confidence, and peace of mind, learn more about our services at www.nursing-hometrusts.org.

What Happens When You Visit www. nursinghometrusts.org?

First, you'll notice the "How Much Can I Protect?" button on our site. That button will take you to an estimator that calculates how much you can protect by following the strategies in this book. It takes only five minutes.

Once you get your protection estimate, we'll invite you to book a free consultation with one of our licensed representatives. During that call, we'll let you know in exact terms how we can help you. It may take only a digital signature on some paperwork that costs you nothing.

If you're in crisis planning mode and your loved one is already in a nursing home, spending down is necessary right now. Depending on how many children your loved ones have and their total assets, a funeral expense trust for Mom and burial space item trusts for the kids may be enough to spend down completely. Then all the money will be protected when Mom applies for Medicaid. Once she's accepted, you're in the clear.

Maybe your loved one has a home and needs to sell it. Or you have a lot of money, and you want to set up a single premium immediate annuity in conjunction with an elder care attorney. We'll work on that project together and get an attorney in the mix.

Or maybe you're planning well in advance and just need an attorney to establish some trusts. Whatever you need for your current situation, we'll be ready to assist you.

Now is the time to protect your family legacy. Visit www. nursinghometrusts.org and set up your free consultation with us.

GLOSSARY

●

Annuity: a long-term investment issued by an insurance company designed to help protect you from the risk of outliving your income.

Bankruptcy: a legal proceeding for people or businesses that are unable to repay their outstanding debts.

Burial space item: physical items such as caskets, urns, vaults, burial plots, cremation niches, headstones, as well as the opening and closing of the grave and perpetual care of these things. Such items are counted as separate from burial funds.

Common level ratio: the ratio of assessed value to current market value, usually assigned by the county for a given area.

Community spouse: the spouse of an individual receiving Medicaid-funded, long-term care in an institutional setting who does not living in a facility themselves.

Community Spouse Resource Allowance (CSRA): the amount of assets the community spouse is allowed to keep under a state's spousal impoverishment law.

Equity: ownership of assets that may have debts or other liabilities attached to them.

Escrow: an arrangement to have funds held by a third party.

Estate: the collective sum of an individual's net worth, including all property, possessions, and other assets, minus any liabilities owed.

Irrevocable burial space item trust: a trust that can't be used for funeral services but can be used for any burial space items. Medicaid cannot seize the unused portion after the funeral.

Irrevocable estate planning trust: a trust that protects $2,500 to $100,000 tax-free for the trust's beneficiaries following a five-year waiting period and after the trust grantor's death.

Irrevocable funeral expense trust: a trust that covers funeral expenses and doesn't count toward the patient's assets. Medicaid can still seize the unused portion.

Irrevocable income only trust: a trust that allows the recipient to access only the returns (or income) of the assets in it, not the underlying principal.

Irrevocable trusts: trusts where the terms cannot be modified, amended, or terminated without the permission of the grantor's beneficiary or beneficiaries.

Long-term care insurance (LTC): an insurance policy that covers costs when the covered person can no longer perform certain functions for themselves, such as bathing, eating, or cognitive functions.

Look-back period: a five-year period that Medicaid can audit for potential assets, which is used to determine the length of a penalty period.

Medicaid: a federal and state program that helps with health care costs for some people with limited income and resources, including benefits not normally covered by Medicare, such as nursing home care and personal care services.

Medicare: a single-payer national social insurance program in the United States, primarily providing health insurance for Americans ages sixty-five and older but also for some younger people with disabilities.

Penalty divisor: the average cost of private pay nursing home care in the state or region in which one resides. This is used to calculate how many months the Medicaid penalty period lasts.

Penalty period: the number of days Medicaid will wait before paying for care, determined by the amount of assets the patient had during the look-back period divided by the penalty divisor.

Revenue cycle management: the financial process nursing home corporations use to manage payments, focusing specifically on the payment transition between private pay (your dollars) and Medicaid.

Single premium immediate annuity (SPIA): an annuity purchased with a single lump sum that begins paying out either immediately or within a year of purchase.

Snapshot date: the date an individual's spouse is admitted to long-term care; used to calculate the precise look-back period.

Special needs trust: a trust that pays the beneficiary for nonmedical needs not covered by Medicaid, such as nonfood groceries, dental work, clothing, phones, and transportation.

Spend-down period: the period after Medicare benefits lapse where the nursing home will attempt to spend down the patient's assets until they qualify for Medicaid.

Spousal impoverishment law: a federal law (also known as the division of assets) that protects a community spouse by preventing Medicaid from combining the assets and income of both spouses to pay for care, which would leave the community spouse impoverished and unable to support themselves.

Trusts: property interests held by one person for the benefit of another.

Waiver: a program that allows for exemptions from certain regulations in specific circumstances.

Whole life insurance: a type of life insurance that costs the same as long as the insured person is alive and that pays benefits to survivors when the person has died.

APPENDIX: STATE-BY-STATE MEDICAID PLANNING FIGURES

•

State Medicaid planning figures are subject to change throughout the year. Here are the most current figures at the time of publication.

Alabama

Divestment Penalty Divisor:
$6,600 per month
Minimum Community Spouse Resource Allowance:
$27,480
Maximum Community Spouse Resource Allowance:
$137,400
Home Equity Limitation:
$636,000
Funeral Expense Trust Limitation:
$15,000
Source: Medicaid, as of July 2022

Alaska

Divestment Penalty Divisor:
varies by facility
Community Spouse Resource Allowance:
$137,400
Home Equity Limitation:
$636,000

Funeral Expense Trust Limitation:
$1,500
Source: Medicaid, as of January 2022

Arizona

Divestment Penalty Divisor:
$8,029.46 (Maricopa, Pima, and Pinal counties) or $7,331.78 (all others)
Minimum Community Spouse Resource Allowance:
$27,480
Maximum Community Spouse Resource Allowance:
$137,400
Home Equity Limitation:
$636,000
Funeral Expense Trust Limitation:
$9,000 (a letter of G&S may be required)
Source: Medicaid, as of July 2022

Arkansas

Divestment Penalty Divisor:
$7,151
Minimum Community Spouse Resource Allowance:
$27,480
Maximum Community Spouse Resource Allowance:
$137,400
Home Equity Limitation:
$636,000
Funeral Expense Trust Limitation:
$15,000
Source: Medicaid, as of July 2022

California

Divestment Penalty Divisor:
$10,933
Community Spouse Resource Allowance:
$137,400
Home Equity Limitation:
None
Funeral Expense Trust Limitation:
$15,000
Source: Medicaid, as of April 2022

Colorado

Divestment Penalty Divisor:
$8,609
Minimum Community Spouse Resource Allowance:
$2,288.75
Maximum Community Spouse Resource Allowance:
$3,435
Home Equity Limitation:
$955,000
Funeral Expense Trust Limitation:
$15,000
Source: Medicaid, as of July 2022

Connecticut

Divestment Penalty Divisor:
$14,060
Minimum Community Spouse Resource Allowance:
$27,480
Maximum Community Spouse Resource Allowance:
$137,400

Home Equity Limitation:
$955,000
Funeral Expense Trust Limitation:
$10,000
Source: Medicaid, as of July 2022

Delaware

Divestment Penalty Divisor:
$354.91 per day or $10,795 per month
Minimum Community Spouse Resource Allowance:
$27,480
Maximum Community Spouse Resource Allowance:
$137,400
Home Equity Limitation:
$636,000
Funeral Expense Trust Limitation:
$15,000
Source: Medicaid, as of July 2022

District of Columbia

Divestment Penalty Divisor:
$14,175.99
Minimum Community Spouse Resource Allowance:
$27,480
Maximum Community Spouse Resource Allowance:
$137,400
Home Equity Limitation:
$955,000
Funeral Expense Trust Limitation:
$15,000
Source: Medicaid, as of January 2022

Florida

Divestment Penalty Divisor:
$9,703
Minimum Community Spouse Resource Allowance:
$2,288.75
Maximum Community Spouse Resource Allowance:
$3,435
Home Equity Limitation:
$636,000
Funeral Expense Trust Limitation:
$15,000
Source: Medicaid, as of July 2022

Georgia

Divestment Penalty Divisor:
$8,821
Community Spouse Resource Allowance:
$137,400
Home Equity Limitation:
$636,000
Funeral Expense Trust Limitation:
$10,000
Source: Medicaid, as of January 2022

Hawaii

Divestment Penalty Divisor:
$8,850
Community Spouse Resource Allowance:
$137,400
Home Equity Limitation:
$955,000

Funeral Expense Trust Limitation:
   $15,000
Source: Medicaid, as of January 2022

Idaho

Divestment Penalty Divisor:
   $312 per day or $9,481 per month
Minimum Community Spouse Resource Allowance:
   $27,480
Maximum Community Spouse Resource Allowance:
   $137,400
Home Equity Limitation:
   $750,000
Funeral Expense Trust Limitation:
   $15,000
Source: Medicaid, as of July 2022

Illinois

Divestment Penalty Divisor:
   monthly private pay rate
Supportive Living Penalty Divisor:
   $181 per day or $5,430 per month
Community Spouse Resource Allowance:
   $109,560
Home Equity Limitation:
   $636,000
Funeral Expense Trust Limitation:
   $6,562 (without G&S) or $15,000 (with G&S)
Source: Medicaid, as of January 2022

Indiana

Divestment Penalty Divisor:
$7,167
Minimum Community Spouse Resource Allowance:
$27,480
Maximum Community Spouse Resource Allowance:
$137,400
Home Equity Limitation:
$636,000
Funeral Expense Trust Limitation:
$15,000
Source: Medicaid, as of July 2022

Iowa

Divestment Penalty Divisor:
$256.13 per day or $7,786.35 per month
Minimum Community Spouse Resource Allowance:
$27,480
Maximum Community Spouse Resource Allowance:
$137,400
Home Equity Limitation:
$636,000
Funeral Expense Trust Limitation:
$13,125 (without G&S) or $15,000 (with G&S)
Source: Medicaid, as of July 2022

Kansas

Divestment Penalty Divisor:
$234.27 per day
Minimum Community Spouse Resource Allowance:
$27,480

Maximum Community Spouse Resource Allowance:
$137,400
Home Equity Limitation:
$636,000
Funeral Expense Trust Limitation:
$10,000
Source: Medicaid, as of July 2022

Kentucky

Divestment Penalty Divisor:
$252.43 per day
Minimum Community Spouse Resource Allowance:
$27,480
Maximum Community Spouse Resource Allowance:
$137,400
Home Equity Limitation:
$636,000
Funeral Expense Trust Limitation:
$15,000 (a letter of G&S may be required)
Source: Medicaid, as of July 2022

Louisiana

Divestment Penalty Divisor:
$164.38 per day or $5,000 per month
Community Spouse Resource Allowance:
$137,400
Home Equity Limitation:
$636,000
Funeral Expense Trust Limitation:
$10,000
Source: Medicaid, as of January 2022

Maine

Divestment Penalty Divisor:
    $8,476
Community Spouse Resource Allowance:
    $137,400
Home Equity Limitation:
    $955,000
Funeral Expense Trust Limitation:
    $12,000
Source: Medicaid, as of July 2022

Maryland

Divestment Penalty Divisor:
    $350 per day or $10,190 per month
Minimum Community Spouse Resource Allowance:
    $27,480
Maximum Community Spouse Resource Allowance:
    $137,400
Home Equity Limitation:
    $636,000
Funeral Expense Trust Limitation:
    $15,000
Source: Medicaid, as of July 2022

Massachusetts

Divestment Penalty Divisor:
    $410 per day
Minimum Community Spouse Resource Allowance:
    $27,480
Maximum Community Spouse Resource Allowance:
    $137,400

Home Equity Limitation:
$955,000
Funeral Expense Trust Limitation:
$15,000 (a letter of G&S may be required)
Source: Medicaid, as of July 2022

Michigan

Divestment Penalty Divisor:
$9,880
Minimum Community Spouse Resource Allowance:
$27,480
Maximum Community Spouse Resource Allowance:
$137,400
Home Equity Limitation:
$636,000
Funeral Expense Trust Limitation:
not available
Source: Medicaid, as of July 2022

Minnesota

Divestment Penalty Divisor:
$8,781
Community Spouse Resource Allowance:
$137,400
Home Equity Limitation:
$636,000
Funeral Expense Trust Limitation:
$15,000 (a letter of G&S may be required)
Source: Medicaid, as of July 2022

Mississippi

Divestment Penalty Divisor:
$233 per day or $7,107 per month
Community Spouse Resource Allowance:
$137,400
Home Equity Limitation:
$636,000
Funeral Expense Trust Limitation:
$15,000
Source: Medicaid, as of July 2022

Missouri

Divestment Penalty Divisor:
$6,894
Minimum Community Spouse Resource Allowance:
$27,480
Maximum Community Spouse Resource Allowance:
$137,400
Home Equity Limitation:
$636,000
Funeral Expense Trust Limitation:
$9,999 (a letter of G&S may be required)
Source: Medicaid, as of July 2022

Montana

Divestment Penalty Divisor:
$261.53 per day or $7,954.87 per month
Minimum Community Spouse Resource Allowance:
$27,480
Maximum Community Spouse Resource Allowance:
$137,400

Home Equity Limitation:
$636,000
Funeral Expense Trust Limitation:
$15,000
Source: Medicaid, as of July 2022

Nebraska

Divestment Penalty Divisor:
monthly private pay rate
Minimum Community Spouse Resource Allowance:
$27,480
Maximum Community Spouse Resource Allowance:
$137,400
Home Equity Limitation:
$636,000
Funeral Expense Trust Limitation:
$5,654
Source: Medicaid, as of July 2022

Nevada

Divestment Penalty Divisor:
$9,059.10
Community Spouse Resource Allowance:
$137,400
Home Equity Limitation:
$636,000
Funeral Expense Trust Limitation:
$15,000 (a letter of G&S may be required)
Source: Medicaid, as of July 2022

New Hampshire

Divestment Penalty Divisor:
$342.80 per day or $10,427.98 per month
Minimum Community Spouse Resource Allowance:
$27,480
Maximum Community Spouse Resource Allowance:
$137,400
Home Equity Limitation:
$636,000
Funeral Expense Trust Limitation:
$15,000 (a letter of G&S may be required)
Source: Medicaid, as of July 2022

New Jersey

Divestment Penalty Divisor:
$374.39 per day
Minimum Community Spouse Resource Allowance:
$27,480
Maximum Community Spouse Resource Allowance:
$137,400
Home Equity Limitation:
$955,000
Funeral Expense Trust Limitation:
$15,000 (a letter of G&S may be required)
Source: Medicaid, as of July 2022

New Mexico

Divestment Penalty Divisor:
$7,811
Minimum Community Spouse Resource Allowance:
$31,290

Maximum Community Spouse Resource Allowance:
> $137,400

Home Equity Limitation:
> $636,000

Funeral Expense Trust Limitation:
> $15,000

Source: Medicaid, as of July 2022

New York

Divestment Penalty Divisor:
> $11,328 (Central New York)
> $14,012 (Long Island)
> $12,560 (New York City)
> $13,399 (Northeastern New York)
> $13,415 (N. Metropolitan)
> $13,376 (Rochester)
> $11,884 (Western New York)

Minimum Community Spouse Resource Allowance:
> $74,820

Maximum Community Spouse Resource Allowance:
> $137,400

Home Equity Limitation:
> $955,000

Funeral Expense Trust Limitation:
>   not available

Source: Medicaid, as of January 2022

North Carolina

Divestment Penalty Divisor:
> $237 per day or $7,110 per month

Minimum Community Spouse Resource Allowance:
> $27,480

Maximum Community Spouse Resource Allowance:
$137,400
Home Equity Limitation:
$636,000
Funeral Expense Trust Limitation:
$15,000
Source: Medicaid, as of July 2022

North Dakota

Divestment Penalty Divisor:
$352.42 per day or $10,719 per month
Minimum Community Spouse Resource Allowance:
$27,480
Maximum Community Spouse Resource Allowance:
$137,400
Home Equity Limitation:
$636,000
Funeral Expense Trust Limitation:
$6,000
Source: Medicaid, as of January 2022

Ohio

Divestment Penalty Divisor:
$6,905
Minimum Community Spouse Resource Allowance:
$27,480
Maximum Community Spouse Resource Allowance:
$137,400
Home Equity Limitation:
$636,000
Funeral Expense Trust Limitation:
$15,000
Source: Medicaid, as of July 2022

Oklahoma

Divestment Penalty Divisor:
$188.21 per day
Minimum Community Spouse Resource Allowance:
$27,480
Maximum Community Spouse Resource Allowance:
$137,400
Home Equity Limitation:
$636,000
Funeral Expense Trust Limitation:
$10,000
Source: Medicaid, as of January 2022

Oregon

Divestment Penalty Divisor:
$9,551
Minimum Community Spouse Resource Allowance:
$27,480
Maximum Community Spouse Resource Allowance:
$137,400
Home Equity Limitation:
$636,000
Funeral Expense Trust Limitation:
$15,000
Source: Medicaid, as of July 2022

Pennsylvania

Divestment Penalty Divisor:
$482.50 per day or $14,676.04 per month
Minimum Community Spouse Resource Allowance:
$27,480

Maximum Community Spouse Resource Allowance:
$137,400
Home Equity Limitation:
$636,000
Funeral Expense Trust Limitation:
varies by county
Source: Medicaid, as of July 2022

Rhode Island

Divestment Penalty Divisor:
$328 per day or $9,961 per month
Minimum Community Spouse Resource Allowance:
$27,480
Maximum Community Spouse Resource Allowance:
$137,400
Home Equity Limitation:
$636,000
Funeral Expense Trust Limitation:
$15,000
Source: Medicaid, as of July 2022

South Carolina

Divestment Penalty Divisor:
$274.52 per day or $8,349.98 per month
Community Spouse Resource Allowance:
$66,480
Home Equity Limitation:
$636,000
Funeral Expense Trust Limitation:
$15,000
Source: Medicaid, as of January 2022

South Dakota

Divestment Penalty Divisor:
$268.21 per day or $8,158.12 per month
Minimum Community Spouse Resource Allowance:
$27,480
Maximum Community Spouse Resource Allowance:
$137,400
Home Equity Limitation:
$636,000
Funeral Expense Trust Limitation:
$15,000
Source: Medicaid, as of July 2022

Tennessee

Divestment Penalty Divisor:
$228.41 per day or $6,852.30 per month
Minimum Community Spouse Resource Allowance:
$27,480
Maximum Community Spouse Resource Allowance:
$137,400
Home Equity Limitation:
$636,000
Funeral Expense Trust Limitation:
$6,000
Source: Medicaid, as of July 2022

Texas

Divestment Penalty Divisor:
$237.93 per day or $7,212 per month
Minimum Community Spouse Resource Allowance:
$27,480

Maximum Community Spouse Resource Allowance:
$137,400
Home Equity Limitation:
$636,000
Funeral Expense Trust Limitation:
$15,000
Source: Medicaid, as of January 2022

Utah

Divestment Penalty Divisor:
$6,908
Minimum Community Spouse Resource Allowance:
$27,480
Maximum Community Spouse Resource Allowance:
$137,400
Home Equity Limitation:
$636,000
Funeral Expense Trust Limitation:
$7,000
Source: Medicaid, as of July 2022

Vermont

Divestment Penalty Divisor:
$338.28 per day or $10,148.35 per month
Community Spouse Resource Allowance:
$137,400
Home Equity Limitation:
$636,000
Funeral Expense Trust Limitation:
$10,000
Source: Medicaid, as of July 2022

Virginia

Divestment Penalty Divisor:
$9,032 for Northern Virginia (the cities and counties of Alexandria, Arlington, Fairfax, Falls Church, Loudoun, Manassas, Prince William), and $6,422 (all others)
Minimum Community Spouse Resource Allowance:
$27,480
Maximum Community Spouse Resource Allowance:
$137,400
Home Equity Limitation:
$636,000
Funeral Expense Trust Limitation:
$15,000
Source: Medicaid, as of July 2022

Washington

Divestment Penalty Divisor:
$355 per day or $10,785 per month
Minimum Community Spouse Resource Allowance:
$59,890
Maximum Community Spouse Resource Allowance:
$137,400
Home Equity Limitation:
$636,000
Funeral Expense Trust Limitation:
$15,000
Source: Medicaid, as of July 2022

West Virginia

Divestment Penalty Divisor:
$355 per day or $10,650 per month

Minimum Community Spouse Resource Allowance:
$27,480
Maximum Community Spouse Resource Allowance:
$137,400
Home Equity Limitation:
$636,000
Funeral Expense Trust Limitation:
$15,000 (a letter of G&S may be required)
Source: Medicaid, as of July 2022

Wisconsin

Divestment Penalty Divisor:
$307.40 per day or $9,350.08 per month
Minimum Community Spouse Resource Allowance:
$50,000
Maximum Community Spouse Resource Allowance:
$137,400
Home Equity Limitation:
$955,000
Funeral Expense Trust Limitation:
$15,000 (a letter of G&S may be required)
Source: Medicaid, as of January 2022

Wyoming

Divestment Penalty Divisor:
$8,087
Community Spouse Resource Allowance:
$137,400
Home Equity Limitation:
$636,000
Funeral Expense Trust Limitation:
$15,000 (a letter of G&S may be required)
Source: Medicaid, as of January 2022

ACKNOWLEDGMENTS

———————— ● ————————

This book would not exist without the family business, Golden Considerations of Dallastown, Pennsylvania. Bob Rae, my father, founded decades ago what is now the nation's largest independent broker of funeral trust products. Golden Considerations has helped millions navigate with wisdom and care the complexities of end-of-life financial concerns. It's an honor to be in the next generation, Dad.

I'd also like to thank elder care attorney Jeff Bellomo, who has been an invaluable industry partner.

And special thanks to my book coach and editor, Joshua Lisec. He took the information in my head and transformed it into a useful, educational book of which I am proud. Thanks, Joshua!

ABOUT THE AUTHOR

———————— ● ————————

Joshua Rae is vice president of Golden Considerations, the nation's largest independent broker of funeral trust products. Rae helps senior citizens and their families plan for the future and protect their assets from nursing homes, creditors, and probate court. To learn how to protect your life savings for the next generation, visit www.nursinghometrusts.org.

www.ingramcontent.com/pod-product-compliance
Lightning Source LLC
Chambersburg PA
CBHW051728260326
41914CB00040B/2011/J